How to Become the Greatest at Oral Sex 4: Freaky Sex Tips and Sex Tricks

JESSICA KING

ISBN: **1979694435**
ISBN-13: **978-1979694438**

This book is dedicate d to Venus

May she help you find love.

CONTENTS

ACKNOWLEDGMENTS

I would like to take this opportunity to thank my supporters, because of you, I am driven, inspired and committed to producing newer and more profound material that speaks volume to the topics you care so deeply about. Thank you for the privilege of your continued support, it means more to me than you will ever know.

I would also like to thank my friends and family for remaining by my side, and my boyfriend, thank you, too, for your love and unwavering support.

Thank you to the bloggers for the extensive promotions and to the indie publishing world at large for helping me realize this dream, thank you, thank you, thank you.

1 GET YOUR KINK ON

Introduction

I know, you've been dying for some unusual, kinky sex tips to spice up your love life. The wait is over and now it's time to become a master of the bedroom.

Beware, this book is not for the faint of heart. Following this pretty short introduction will be some really extreme stuff. This would require you to completely abandon your comfort zone so you can have mind-blowing sex. If you want to learn some new bedroom tricks but you're a bit prudish then this book will completely transform you. Not up for it? Don't worry there are some tamer guides out there in the big wide world you can check out – they're not as fun though.

Let's say you're willing to take up the challenge and decide to read the entire book. I've got one word for you... Congrats! You're well on your way to becoming a sexy seductive freak that will turn your man's knees to jello. He'll both love and fear fucking you because of the crazy, seductive things you'll be doing to him. You'll have him wrapped around your finger forever.

This topic has become a passion of mine because of how it can positively transform lives and relationships. Much of these I draw from experiences and just to make sure you get comprehensive advice I've consulted with numerous sex experts (sexperts as I like to call them). Now that you're fully committed to becoming a badass in bed let's fill your bag with tricks.

Crotchless panties

And here you thought lacy panties were badass? Any woman who wants to give her man's eyes something to feast on usually have a pair of lingerie or two tucked away for special occasions. But it's time turn up the heat in your bedroom with a new level of sexy.

Nothing says kinky as fuck like crotchless panties.

It's hard to imagine that at one point in time these were openly welcomed in the bedroom. However, they were soon seen as too exotic and were damned to live out the rest of their lives in strip clubs and on escorts. Well, now we're going to turn your bedroom into a private strip club so you can escort your man to sensual orgasms.

Tiana Reid, one of our sexperts, confirms that crotchless panties rank among the highest things banished from the bedroom. However, we're looking to destroy this stigma surrounding these huge turn-ons. You must adopt an open mind. Get excited about trying new experiences like this. Think about it, the only risk you face is your man's boner busting through his pants.

Tiana explains: "Crotchless panties are insanely hot. Just looking at them screams 'I don't care where just give it to me!'. Your man will get an instant hard-on that he won't have trouble putting inside you.

"When it comes to crotchless style panties I recommend choosing one with a tight elastic that frames the exposed area. It will increase the sensitivity by putting more pressure on the outer lips of the vagina."

Pinwheels

Ever accidentally pricked a pin on your finger? Yeah, it hurts like hell. Since it's so painful only a crazy woman would do it on purpose, right? Well as counterintuitive as it sounds, Tiana explains that this pin trick can be really hot – no pun intended.

Hey, if it's your first time playing with pin penetration we advise to take it slow. Start with something more manageable like pinwheels.

"When you first think about it, you're bound to talk yourself out right away. But if you pursue it, you'll get a wild experience that stimulates your mind and nerves."

I understand, if you're new to it, it's going to seem scary at first; you might even back out. But here's why you should try it out. Touch sensations often add another level of intensity to sex. I'm sure your woman-parts jump whenever your man touches you in the right spot. Adding a different type of sensation like pins in just the right way can be deeply pleasurable and send you into an erotic overdrive. You'll be surprised at how good it feels.

Tiana says: "Best one to use when getting into this is the crave rose gold pinwheel and razor tool. It looks and feels great and won't be too intimidating for newbies. Run the wheel over sensitive areas such as nipples with light pressure until your partner adjusts to the sensation."

Just a heads up from wise fools who suffered from trial and error. Do it sober and conscious. Never when you're drunk, distracted or high. Not even if you're *just* tipsy. You have to be really focused. One mistake and instead of having a great time your lover ends up in the ER trying to explain the entire situation.

"Pay attention to how your partner reacts to everything you do. The pinwheel is great to explore new sensations and bring you two closer, just be careful with your strokes," she adds.

Crop it

This is for those of you who have a secret interest in domination. If you want to try it out, then the best place to start is with a good crop. No, not food, that part comes later. Here's what Tiana advises,

"Getting a crop must've have crossed your mind several times if you like a little domination. With the crack of a whip, your man will be obeying you're every order."

It's not just about the kinkiness of domination. Sex utilizes all your senses and the crop emphasize on sounds and feel. He'll clench in anticipation when he hears the crack of the whip. Once the leather stings his bare skin the pain will feel pleasurable since all his tense muscles will relax. All these sensations will make him erupt with carnal energy. The only caution, consider moderation.

"Turn it up by blindfolding him. The sounds will have an entirely different effect."

Go ginger

They say redheads are pretty freaky in bed. Increase your freakiness with another layer of ginger by rubbing it all over your body.

Tiana says: "The world is waking up to ginger's many health benefits and now you'll be adding a sexual one as well.

"It'll create a bewildering tingling feeling on the skin which gets more intense when applied to sensitive areas. Just be cautious with where you put it.

"Cut it up in big chunks with the skin still attached in some places for you to safely grip.

"Get started by rubbing gently around the nipples and then slowly move to the genitals. Again be very attentive to your partner's reactions. Take your time to avoid overwhelming sensations."

Electricity

Whenever someone uses the phrase "sparks fly" when two people get together I'm sure they weren't thinking of this next sex tip. Though you've never even considered using electricity in such a way you might discover how much more interesting it makes things. And don't worry you won't electrocute anyone.

Tiana says electricity excites a unique erotic feeling within us.

"People don't often consider messing with electricity in the bedroom. But once they discover Coco de Mer's ElectraStim, it'll change their perspectives. You can use all sorts of regular toys along with the modified ones to get the most pleasure."

"Newbies to electric toys should start with the electric pads. Once you've secured them to yourself and your partner you can have an electrifying time."

Weighty dildos

Dildos aren't really a topic many are comfortable with and can lead to horrible imaginations.

However, Trudy says it's best to ditch that mindset

and be more open-minded about trying weighty Dildos.

"People tend to be afraid of dildos but once they get one that suits them it becomes their best friend. Steel and glass dildos are especially geared towards increasing sensations since it's easier to press against the front of the vagina"

Trying these will definitely up your kink factor and pleasure.

Anal stimulators for her

Anal play is a touchy topic for some couples while others have been considering it but haven't really done anything. For those of you who have anal at the top of your lists we'll show you the right way to do it – surprisingly it's not as simple as it sounds.

Trudy informs us that butt plugs are double the fun since they excite your partner just as much as you.

"A fairly big butt plug will increase your pleasure since it encourages the penis to press against the G spot

"Alternatively a pointed one will massage his penis as he thrusts. Both will result in a great orgasm," she says.

2 ANAL STIMULATION

There's no way you can dive into anal without being comfortable first. Both your mind and your body needs to be at ease to enjoy the sensations. This means you should be patient when dealing with something like this. We recommend that you take some time to become "familiar" with it by yourself first. This way there won't be any external pressure from your lover or anyone around you. You won't have to fake feeling good or hit them on reflex when they don't poke you right. Take it slowly by yourself first. Figure out what you like and don't like. Then it'll be easier when your lover come's around. If on the other hand, you're perfectly comfortable with trying things with your partner present then that's fine too. Once you feel at ease and the situation feels right then go for it.

The two keys to anal fun are lubricant and patience. Starting off anal stuff with something like a massage is advisable. Play with the senses to relax and get in the mood. The anus is a ring of muscle. Being completely relaxed will make the entire thing a lot smoother. It's important that you let your partner know that once things get too painful or uncomfortable then it's time to stop. To ensure that you have the best experience we have prepared guidelines that you can follow.

Fingering is usually a go-to move when it comes to anal play. However, sticking to just that will limit the fun you can have. Adding toys to the mix will make things better. You can try these anal toys:

Butt Plugs

Butt plugs are specifically designed to help the anal muscles adjust to being stretched beyond what it's accustomed to. Since it's unnoticeable it can be fun for couples who love public experimentation.

There are a diverse collection of butt plugs to choose from that won't drain your pockets. We recommend anything that's made by LELO and FunFactory. They make long lasting products that are safe to use and perfect for beginners. To sample their bests, in terms of quality and design, you can try the FunFactory Bootie and nJoy Pure Plug.

Anal Beads

Somewhat like prayer beads for worshipping the butt, anal beads should be inserted into your butt one at a time. There's an unexplainable satisfaction that many people experience as their bodies re-adjust to each bead. To increase this sensation most beads are made with beads that gradual increase in diameter. Don't worry about anything getting stuck though, they can all be pulled out with a small handle.

To be on the safe side, always make sure that the beads you use are of the highest quality and pretty durable. The last thing you want is to find yourself having to explain your embarrassing situation to doctors who want to relieve your suffering. For this, we recommend the FunFactory Felix. Newbies will enjoy it since it's usually smaller in diameter compared to others on the market. In light of this, once the beads are pure silicone, flexible and sized for beginners it should get the job done.

Anal Dildos

The only difference between these and vaginal dildos is basically where you put them. It's a perfect starting point for couples who want to explore anal sex. Many people use it to experience a kind of fullness inside them.

Though it may sound very simple, there's ample consideration that needs to be put in on your part. Such things include making sure the dildo has a large base that's easy to hold when removing. You don't want it slipping in too far and you end up in the emergency room a second time. Also be mindful of the dildo's diameter. Newbies should use anything between 0.75" and 1.5". One of the well-known choices you can get your hands on is the Tantus Silk line toys.

Prostate Massagers

Many open-minded men usually dig this stuff since it stimulates the prostate from within the butt. Most of these gadgets have designs similar to dildos but others are completely hands-free. Ones like the latter utilize flexing the muscles to massage the toy into the prostate. As a pleasure bonus, some of these also have nubs to hit more sensitive parts.

If you prefer a firmer approach, Aneros is famous for making massagers of this kind of build. They're among the top prostate massager manufacturers who build their products from rigid materials that stroke the prostate firmly.

To progress adeptly in anal pleasure it's best to get a beginner's kit that has a multitude of tools and toys. Some toys may even come in different sizes so you can increase or decrease depending on your comfort level.

Despite the approach you may take as your "gateway drug" to anal pleasure exploring them will provide you with new and exciting ways to feel great.

3 FREAKY ANAL SEX POSITIONS

Anal sex positions

Anal sex – voodoo for some and exotic adventure for others. Not everyone has the same stance on this kind of sex, but if you're open to it then we have some great positions for you. No pun intended.

Pornstars are fans of having anal sex in the common doggy style position. But remember, they are actors. So even if the pain is killing them they'll act like their having the time of their lives. For those of you who aren't used to it, starting off in doggy will hurt like hell if you don't prepare accordingly.

Jodi Fraser, another one of our sexperts and also relationship guru, has some great tips for us. She knows the best positions that'll make you scream OMG.

She advises that you must be mindful that anal sex is completely different from vaginal intercourse. This means you would need to be more careful and prepared for the task.

"Take an approach that gets both of you ready for anal sex so nothing weird happens. This means exploring around and with the anus to take note of the body's response to stimulation. The next step is relaxing the body with a massage that would mostly be centered around the buttocks spreading outwards. Once the tension is relieved, start playing with anal sex toys like butt plugs and vibrators.," she says.

To make sure you actually enjoy anal sex don't be stingy with foreplay or lube. Now that you're warmed up it's time to use some fantastic positions.

The Curled Angel

Jodi recommends beginning with the spoon position since it's naturally a relaxed one. With your man lying behind you bend your bodies together so you're a bit curled up. From here he can also stimulate other sensitive areas like your clit and breasts.

Jodi says: "Starting with this position is great since it allows the woman to widen her external sphincter for easier penetration. She can simply by stretching her bent legs away from her body."

The Double Decker

This is what happens when you flip the spoon on its back – so to speak. The Double Decker position is transitioning from the Spoon by flipping over to have your bodies face upward.

The intimate closeness is still maintained with this unique position.

Additionally, with you on top, you have a lot more control of the pace and depth of the strokes for maximum

stimulation. As long as he doesn't mind basing your body
he'll enjoy it too.

Afternoon Delight

This is your go-to position when spooning gets a bit old
to you.

In Afternoon Delight your partner is in the same
position but you're back will be at a 90-degree angle.
Since your anus is a bit wider in this position he can just
slide in with minimal effort.

He can also play with your sensitive parts, and you can
Massage his balls too.

The Clip

Being on top may take some extra effort on your part
but it's always worth it. From this vantage point your
partner will get an eye full of all your curves and if Jodi
says you have a higher chance of an orgasm in this
position there's nothing stopping you from trying it out.

This position has the advantage of increasing pleasure
once you arch your back away from him.

Jodi says: "Since women on top positions give her the
ability to make adjustments that intensify clitoral
stimulation. This position will stretch the skin of the anus
which also pulls on the clitoris."

The Rocking Horse

The anus is a very sensitive area and needs to be
approached with caution. When engaging in anal sex
applying the right pressure and depth is the difference
between pleasure and pain. As with other on top

positions, this one gives you more control so you can enjoy the ride more.

To get The Rocking Horse Right, have your man sit with his legs crossed and lean back to keep himself balanced as you straddle him.

As you grind on him this will stimulate your clitoris and allows for some sexy pillow talk.

Reverse Cowgirl

This is a common anal sex position for good reasons. It allows you take him as deep, fast or slow as you like. He'll also have a great time watching your ass bounce on his dick.

Never neglect the added impact your fingers can have on each other's bodies. Find the spots that increase pleasure for both of you.

With your man lying down, put his legs together, face away from him, bend your legs and then straddle him. Now show off your riding skills.

The Amazon

Sometimes to have a great experience you need to add something extra. One way we highly suggest is using props.

This is a nice position to spice up your sex life without the neck-breaking angles. You also have more control and it sets you up for a quick orgasm.

It can get so good that you'll lose control of your legs but try your best to stay anchored.

4 FREAKY MUST TRY SEX POSITIONS

1. Inverted Missionary

I'm sure you've heard of missionary mostly through jokes of how boring it is. To escape that boringness, the Inverted Missionary was born.

Make your man lie flat on his back and then you sit on top of him facing his toes. Once he has penetrated you, lean forward and while using your hands as support push your legs back.

2. Froggie Style

Just from the name Froggie style you can guess that it is somewhat like the famous doggy style. The difference is that you squat like a frog instead of getting down on your knees.

Once you're on the floor like you're playing leapfrog, tilt your head forward but keep most of your weight on your legs. Your man can kneel behind you to insert his dick and make gentle strokes.

3. The Yogi

The Yogi is basically an upside down doggy style. If you're tired of suffocating in a pillow or having your neck craned at an uncomfortable angle, then this position is for.

Start by lying flat on the floor or any other alternative surface. Then arch your back as you push off the floor with your hands – somewhat like a yoga wheelbarrow.

The man then enters from a kneeling position between your legs where he can thrust. Recommended for the fittest of us.

4. The Lap Dance

A very easy position you see on Tv and every strip club.

Have your man sit on the edge of the bed, couch or chair. If he needs to, he can rest on his hands behind him for support.

Now go ahead and sit on top of him while facing away. This position is ideal for bouncing or twerking and you can ride as well

5. The Cowpoke

Maybe it's about the badass nature of the wild west days that makes women go head over heels for the cowboy. Most city girls may not agree but they'll definitely love this position. Feel free to roleplay with this one, adding hats, spurs and anything else that makes it sexier.

Have your man lie on his back and pull his legs up to his chest. You can now crouch over him (facing away) and rest on his legs just a bit. Don't put too much pressure or you'll break something.

This is ideal for men with a longer shaft.

6. The Circus Freak

If you're freakishly flexible, then you can use this
position to show off your talent.

This is a standing position so get your partner up and in
front of you. Depending on the height difference you
made need a stool, but that's usually for him. If you're
shorter it'll be even more impressive and sexy. Imagine
splitting while standing.

Now go ahead and raise one leg up to his shoulder,
resting on it lightly. He should be able to further support
you and keep you balanced by holding your waist. From
here he can thrust deep inside you (especially if you're
really flexible)

5 THE GREATEST SEX POSITIONS KNOWN TO MAN

SEX POSITION: THE CAT
a.k.a. Coital Alignment Technique

This technique is great because it results in a lot of clitoral stimulation. A study in the Journal of Sex and Marital therapy suggests that women who had trouble orgasming in the Missionary position had a 56 percent increase in actually orgasming using the Coital Alignment Technique (CAT). That means that they had orgasmed 56% more than usual!

CAT is a slight variation of the missionary. Instead of you and your partner's chests aligning, your man can put his chest closer to your shoulders. Now bend your legs at a 45-degree angle and tilt your hips up. This will but the base of his shaft in a position where it's always massaging your clitoris.

Additionally, you can straighten your legs, have him push his pelvis down a bit while you push up.

Here's a great tip for even more pleasure.

Instead of him thrusting up and down he can rock back and forth to stimulate you enough so you can orgasm quicker. Increase your orgasm even more by making him rotate his pelvis while inside you.

SEX POSITION: WATERFALL
a.k.a. Head Rush

By its nickname, it'll make blood rush to both of his heads.

Make your man move closer to the edge of the bed and lie back with his head on the floor. Get on top, ride him, bounce and do whatever to make him bust. When he orgasms, the blood rushing to his head will create a wicked mind-blowing sensation.

SEX POSITION: ONE UP
a.k.a. Over Your Shoulder, The Hamstring Stretch

This position is ideal for women that tend to have extreme sensitivity, or greater sensitivity, on one side of the clitoris.

Lie on the edge of the bed and have your man kneel on the floor in front of you. Raise one of your legs and keep it up by wrapping your hand around the hamstring area (just below the knee). You can now raise one of your hips slightly to move in unison with his strokes.

To make sure you guys are in sync with perfect rhythm, she can twist a bit. (For more oral sex tips, check out How to Become the Greatest at Oral Sex: Sex secrets that puts a Spell on Him)

Extra Tip For Her

Make it easier for him to pleasure you by demonstrating on his earlobe. Use your tongue to give him an idea of the technique and pressure you prefer.

Extra Tip For Him

While giving her head, follow up your tongue strokes with the knuckle of your fingers. The textural difference between the softness of your tongue and the roughness of your knuckle will evoke a unique, pleasing sensation,

SEX POSITION: THE COWGIRL
a.k.a. Woman On Top

This position gives you more control of your orgasm as it allows you to steer him towards your G-spot for maximum stimulation.

The Cowgirl is one of the best positions out there since it opens her up to various stimulating sensations. In addition to increasing intimacy as you both lock eyes with each other, being in control in this position makes her feel more involved as a sexual partner instead of a sex doll that her man has his way with. Make the most of this position by alternating between shallow and deep thrusts. Shallow thrusts will stimulate the most sensitive parts of her vagina.

Spice things up by lying chest to chest with your legs stretched out on top of his. Brace your feet on top of his and push off for a rocking motion. This will cause some friction between your clitoral area and his pubic bone for more pleasure. (Learn more about her body—and what to do with it—with How to Become the Greatest at Oral Sex 2: The Practical Guide.)

Extra Tip For Him

Make her climax quicker by stimulating her with your fingers or tongue until she's really aroused. Coming from the woman on top position she can squat over your face where you can treat her to a nice head.

SEX POSITION: THE HOT SEAT
a.k.a. The Love Seat, The Man Chair

This one really fires up the G-Spot

Have your man sit on the edge of the bed or on a chair with his feet planted firmly on the floor. Turn away from him and sit between his legs instead of directly on them. In this position, you can ride back and forth using the chair arms as support or push off with your feet. Utilize your ability to control the angle of how he penetrates you by arching your back and pressing your ass into his groin.

Spice things up by reaching under to stimulate his balls, the base of his penis and wherever else he likes. He can also take advantage of the position by playing with your nipples.

Extra Tip For Him

When you know she's not really in the mood for sex gently persuade her by preparing a bubble bath with scented oils, give her a nice massage and ultimately something's   gonna   slip   in.

23

SEX POSITION: SPIN CYCLE
a.k.a. Maytag Repair Man

This one shakes things up a bit.

This is a wild variation of the Hot Seat. You'll still be sitting in your man's lap, but this time you'll both be on top of a washing machine with the agitator cycle maxed out.

SEX POSITION: STAIRWAY TO HEAVEN
a.k.a. Step Lively

Can't wait until you reach the bedroom, this one keeps her steady while you take her on the way there.

This is another variation of the Hot Seat. This time you're sitting on him while he's sitting on the stairs. The handrails will offer you extra support and make it easy for you to lift yourself.

SEX POSITION: REVERSE COWGIRL
a.k.a. Rodeo Drive, Half Way Around the World

The best thing about this position is that your man will get an awesome view of your ass while you control how deep he gets inside you.

Have your man lie on his back with his legs outstretched. Turn away from him and then straddle his hips. From here you can ride and bounce on his penis. If you want even more stimulation, lean forward or backward to change the angle of penetration.

Extra Tip For Her

Since he may have a hard time reaching your sensitive parts in this position go ahead and play with your clit for more pleasure.

SEX POSITION: POLE POSITION
a.k.a. Thighmaster

This one will stimulate multiple areas for you and give your man a nice view of the action.

Have your partner lie on his back and bend a single leg upwards while the other is fully stretched. Now straddle his raised leg, with your thighs hugging his and sit on his penis with your back facing him. Use his knee as support while rocking up and down.

In this position, you can rub your vulva along his thigh to your liking.

Extra Tip For Her

This position gives you the ability to massage his leg and thigh which will be a real treat if he's sensitive in that area. Additionally you can reach other sections of his man parts that he likes to be tended.

For more sex positions, as well as other ways to reignite the passion, check out How to Become the Greatest at Oral Sex 2: The Practical Guide.

SEX POSITION: FACE OFF
a.k.a. The Lap Dance

This is a very intimate position that's ideal for long sessions due to its comfortable arrangement.

Once your partner is sitting on a chair or the edge of the bed, face him, wrap your arms around his back and climb onto his penis. Now that you're comfortably seated you can ride up and down his shaft by using your legs or knees. He can speed up your bounces by grabbing your ass and lifting you.

Make it a whole lot more interesting by using a rocking chair. Old wooden rockers will add a vintage vibe to the whole situation.

Extra Tip For Him

Go for her other erogenous zones like her neck, lips, ears, and nipples. Be creative with how you stimulate these parts of her.

SEX POSITION: THE LAZY MAN
a.k.a. The Squat Thrust

Another position where you're in control while still maintaining deep intimacy.

Make your partner sit on the bed with pillows behind his back for support. Straddle his waist and plant your feet into the bed. Now bend into a squat and slide onto his penis while guiding it with your hand. You can use the balls of your feet to raise or lower self on his shaft as quickly or as slowly as you want to.

Change things up by both of you lying back into the Spider position or Th X if you're experts.

SEX POSITION: DAVID COPPERFIELD

a.k.a. Trick & Treat

If you love strong, upward strokes then this position is perfect for you.

Support your hips with a firm pillow so pelvis is always tilted upwards. Now bend your knees and put your feet on your partner's shoulders.

To make you go wild with pleasure your partner can use a secret sleight of hand trick. While he's stroking you with his tongue direct one of his hands to push upwards on your abdomen. This will cause your skin to stretch from your pubic bone and reveal the head of the clitoris from under the hood. From here he can stimulate the head directly and the sensation will drive you crazy.

Extra Tip For Him

Press your tongue flat against her entire vagina and let her grind on it. She'll naturally fall into a rhythm that will give her maximum arousal. Just don't motorboat it.

SEX POSITION: HEIR TO THE THRONE
a.k.a. Lazy Girl

This is a quick oral sex position that can be done basically anywhere to get you in the mood.

Sit on a chair with your legs wide open. From here your partner can direct the rest of the movie. You can use this position to start your sex session with gentle strokes or bring it to an explosive end with powerful sucking.

If you want a bit of variety, you can use a swivel chair. Try spinning it left and right while keeping your tongue in place.

Extra Tip For Him

Implement a little fingering using your index and ring fingers. Directly stimulate her G-spot by gently stroking the roof of her vagina in a "come here motion". Use your tongue or another hand to apply pressure to her pubic bone. If this double stimulation is done just right, it'll send her over the edge.

SEX POSITION: CLOSED FOR BUSINESS
This is a variation of the One Up that's ideal for slow build-ups.

For some women, direct clitoral stimulation may be uncomfortable. Whether or not this may affect you it's an interesting position to try. With your man's head down on you, loosely close your leg around him. From here he places a hand on your pubic bone while stroking the area around your clit.

Extra Tip For Him

This is another position where you can use the contrasting textures of your tongue and knuckle for a unique sensation.

SEX POSITION: THE PRETZEL
a.k.a. The Pretzel Dip, The Camel Ride

The best thing about this position is that it mixes the deep penetration of doggy style with the intimacy and ease of missionary.

Lie on your left side with your man straddling your left leg. Bend your right leg around the right side of his waist so he can enter you freely. If being entered from behind usually hurts then this position will be a relief. You'll be able to enjoy deep penetration while lying pretty comfortably. Let your partner manually stimulate you with his fingers or rub the head of his penis on your clit. He can do this until your close to orgasm and then he goes back to stroking inside of you.

Extra Tip For Her

Let him know when to go faster, slower, lighter or harder.

Extra Tip For Him

Take it easy at first. Her clitoris is a lot more sensitive than your penis. Doing it too fast or hard at first may end up hurting her. Start gently, then gradually increase speed and pressure.

SEX POSITION: THE G-WHIZ
a.k.a. The Shoulder Holder, The Anvil

This position is good for deep penetration and hits the G-Spot just right.
Lie on your back and have your man kneel between your legs. Lift your legs onto his shoulders and allow him to slide into you. Now he can rock your body side-to-side or up and down so his penis is in constant contact with the front wall of your vagina. Since he's going to be deep

inside you advise him to thrust slowly at first after which he can go faster as you expand to accommodate him.

If you want to be in more control of the rhythm and how deep he goes then move your legs from his shoulders to his chest. With your knees still bent, place your feet flat on his chest and use them to direct his strokes.

Extra Tip For Him

Pay attention to her body to know when she's close to an orgasm. Listen to her breath for when it gets short and shallow. More often than not her skin will flush and her breasts will slightly swell or get larger to signify the climax of her arousal.

SEX POSITION: MAN'S BEST FRIEND
a.k.a. Doggy-Style

The best position for deep penetration and giving your man a great view of your ass.

It's easy, and recommended, to transition into this position from The Flatiron position. While you're on all fours your man can enter from behind and thrust deep. This will allow his penis to touch your cervix. You don't want him banging away at it like a mad dog from the start since it'll hurt a lot. Let him start with slow shallow strokes and then work into slow deep strokes. Once you're accustomed to the rhythm and depth he can bang as hard as you like.

Extra Tip For her

You can increase his orgasm by pushing outward as if you were squeezing him out of your vagina. This causes your vaginal walls to hug his penis for more friction and pleasure. Additionally, it will make your G-Spot more accessible to him so you can feel good too.

6 SPELLBINDING TANTRIC SEX

I'm sure you've heard all the erotic legends of tantric sex. The endless sex sessions, massages that send you on a trip and meditation techniques that turn your squirts into eruptions. This all sounds like it's only achievable by sex gods not mere mortals like ourselves. Can we really profit from tantric sex the way they do?

In fact, yes, and that's what this chapter is all about. Everyone wants longer, more intimate sex that leaves them in a trance. Tantric sex is your ticket to that dream and here's how you can purchase it.

Firstly, I'm going to give you a basic idea of what Tantric sex is.

The tantric journey begins with changing how you view great sex. Tantric sex replaces the boring, in-and-out sprint with a marathon of steamy experiences. While regular sex is all about the climax, tantric sex sidesteps that. It's more about feeding all your sexual senses for a natural orgasm of pure ecstasy.

Most couples find it hard to maintain long periods of meditation and abstinence which are pivotal to tantric sex. We found a way where you can get all the benefits without putting in so much effort.

I've collaborated with Tantric Sex expert Amanda Davids so we could give you the best tips about tantric sex.

Our first technique is just two words.

Eye contact.

You might think you do it all the time but we aren't talking about plain eye contact here. Focused eye contact intensifies the sexual experience for both of you. There's a reason they say the eyes are the windows to the soul. Passionately lock eyes with your partner and you will re-connect on a deeper level. In that space, arousal will amplify as your souls find each other.

Amanda says: "The fastest way to increase intimacy is to capture each other's eyes." As mentioned before, there's a whole lot more to this than just looking. Your gaze must burn with passion and desire.

"Sit together in a spot you won't be disturb. Turn off your phones and other devices so there are no distractions. Close your eyes and center yourself.

"Once you're both ready, open your eyes and look at each other. Let your gaze penetrate beyond what you see and open up yourself to be explored," says Rebecca.

It will feel a bit silly at first, awkward even, but don't stop. Amanda assures us that it's the first phase and once you get past that it will be easier and feel more natural.

"Use this technique during foreplay or incorporate it into a daily routine. Not only does it make sex more intense, it deepens the romance between you two," she says.

Conscious touch

Tantra has a lot of focus on exploring your sexual senses through teasing and building sexual tension. A great way to do that is through touch.

Every single touch must have an intention behind it, none is wasted. Amanda emphasizes that what really gets the magic working is being in the moment.

"Your touch will feel empty and distant if your mind is on other things, like that person who pissed you off at work. If your partner feels that, it's a huge turn off for them," she says.

We get it, being in the right mindset for sex can be difficult. Stress, fatigue and a generally hectic life tend to cause that. But using these techniques will increase your desire for sex as well as the quality of sex. So you end up getting a lot more of the best sex of your life.

Amanda says to put everything in a "Later Box" inside your mind. Shove every worry and distraction in that box and put in the farthest corner of your mind. Don't open it until you're done with your partner. Now all your attention should be on your them and the present moment.

There needs to be a deep desire in your touch. A passionate longing that's translated into each stroke which your partner will feel radiate through their entire body. With such emotions surging through their body, how can they not reach an unparalleled level of satisfaction?

"Be very mindful of where your hands go and the thoughts you hold in your mind as you put them there."

Explore your senses

Unlike ordinary sex, Tantra isn't just about physical intercourse. The power of Tantra comes from the emotional and sensory experience too – this means taste, touch, sight, smell, and sound. These elements are magnified in focus, leading to a new realm of pleasure and ecstasy.

"It's well known that the loss of one sense will gradually heighten others," says Rebecca.

Use this fact to your advantage so you can intensify you and your partner's sexual experiences. Amanda encourages that you focus on individual senses and explore them fully.

"The aim is to cultivate an environment that accentuates your partner's sexual experience. Take away their sight using a blindfold and use a number of things to stimulate their senses.

"For smell, use scents of cinnamon or vanilla. If they're a music lover play their favorite song or something that would really turn them on. If they love words, then read a lyrical love poem. Tantalize their taste buds by feeding them sweet fruits, snacks, and food.

"Explore their sense of touch by using soft fabric such as silk and velvet. Once you've done all of those senses, remove the blindfold and look at them with deep affection and desire."

It will seem like a long process at first but the exotic experience will be worth it.

Full body orgasm

Asking you if you'd like the idea of a full body orgasm would be as ridiculous as asking if you'd want a one-month vacation. We know you'd love it so Amanda will help make it happen.

"You can start having full body orgasms by building up erotic sensations near to your climax and then letting it fade a little.

Then you build it back up again and spread the erotic energy through your entire body. Repeat this for a while. It'll get better and better each time," she says.

So you basically bring them to the brink of orgasm but don't let them actually climax.

"The moment you actually allow yourself to orgasm it will ripple throughout your entire body."

Enjoy the journey

Tantric sex doesn't only focus on orgasms. The fact that the techniques involve delaying orgasms should hint that it's about experiencing a higher level of sexual awareness.

Amanda says some of us will get bored if we put too much emphasis on specific end instead of enjoying the trip there. Tantric sex removes that pressure of only orgasming and increases the fun of sex by ten folds.

"Couples who end up chasing orgasms usually resort to such routines because they're bored with their usual sex. They already know what works and how to get there.

"Take a moment to remember why you love having sex and what it does that makes you look forward to it. Once these are identified, magnify them while exploring other areas you'll both love," says Rebecca.

It could be the intimacy, oral sex, kissing that sends sparks through your body or anything else that excites you. Explore it and then go from there.

7 TIPS AND TRICKS TO MAKE HIM BETTER AT ORAL SEX

Oral sex is usually lumped with other foreplay activities like kissing and stroking, However, it's more intense than those two and we recommend warming up before he goes down on you. We know men get aroused much faster than women do and once they're hard they're tempted to start pleasuring you the moment you hit the sheets. That's all well and good but you can both benefit if you delay him for a little while to replace plundering with caressing, licking and dirty talk.

2. Don't let him pounce on your clit from the get-go. Instead, encourage him to explore everything around your womanhood first as a little tease for the main course. Make him breathe hot and heavy through your underwear and try to suck his way through it before removing them. Direct him to your inner thighs so he can lick, kiss and massage them. Now he can go back up to the pubic area and work his way to the ultimate target.

3. We all desire soft touches in the beginning of oral sex but the more aroused we get the more we want the pressure to be turned up a bit. It's hard for men to read our minds and know just when we want them to revisit moves that were at first uncomfortable. Help him out a little, as well as yourself, and egg him on with what he's doing well and lump in your special request. Say stuff like. "That feels great baby. You know I like it soft don't you.". If you want it harder scream in delight, whisper his name. Adding your moans is all the encouragement he needs to please you just how you like it.

4. Don't zone out just because you're lying back quite relaxed as he does most of the work. There's a lot you can still do to keep engaged in the session. Many women go wild with the idea of grinding against their partner's mouth. Take hold of his head, firmly press it against your vagina, and twist in whatever motion turns you on.

5. During oral sex, most men attempt to penetrate women the same way they would with their penis. Unsurprisingly, this doesn't have the same effect they think it would have. Take the initiative to guide him on how to best please without making it feel like scolding. You can do this by giving him an intense blowjob (tips can be found in How to Become the Greatest at Oral Sex 2: The Practical Guide). But before you start, tell him to give you feedback as you go. He can present a number between 1-10 on how good a certain move feels. Once he's down on you, have him do the same thing.

6. You can make it easier for him to get to your G-Spot by putting a pillow under your ass. This also makes it easier for you to grind your hips on him so it feels great.

7. Sometimes for you to really enjoy oral he would have to put some fingers inside you to stroke your G-Spot. You can direct his hand there or encourage him by saying. "Yeah baby, just like that. Finger me too, I love it."

8. Turn up the intensity by throwing a vibrator into the mix. Let him know that sticking it inside you while he eats you out has always been a long time fantasy of yours.

9. The best thing about normal sex is the feeling of someone's hot, sweaty body slipping across your own. This skin-to-skin action is missing during oral sex and you may end up feeling neglected in certain tender areas. In circumstances like these, you can touch yourself while he works down below. When he looks up and sees how turned on you are it will definitely make him harder. Between your hands and his, you can massage your breasts, stroke your neck and suck on his fingers. You can also put one of your legs against his to feel his erection.

10. Make oral sex more exciting by switching up the positions you use. We all know 69 is a common try-out but how about flipping it on its side. You get on top to sit on his mouth, lean forward and backward or even take your business on the floor where it'll be easier for you move your hips as it provides more support.

11. Love oral sex yet? You should since it offers some crazy intense experiences. The only thing we need to work on is getting it all the time. When he starts talking about sex just say something like this, "It feels so good when you go down on me. You make me come so fast it's insane. We should do it again tonight."

He won't be able to resist giving you the ultimate experience.

8 MORE TIPS AND TRICKS

Oral Sex Tips: How to Become the Greatest at Oral Sex 2: The Practical Guide.

SUPER SLOW & SENSUAL

When it comes to oral, going slow has a potency many wouldn't expect. You can exponentially boost his pleasure by deliberately delaying his climax. It will cause a build-up that leads him to have an explosive orgasm and heavier load. So instead of doing it the way you usually do, slow down your movements to a crawl – to the extent it seems like you're not moving at all.

This will have a weird effect on him that he's not used to and will make you more alluring. It shows a more sensual side of you and as he feels your lips and tongue slowly move over every part of his shaft it will excite him like nothing else. This is especially useful for men who suffer from premature ejaculation.

Super slow means moving no faster than a snail. Kiss, lick and suck him as if you were shot by a slow-mo gun.

WET & SLOPPY

Sloppy, wet head gives a very smooth feeling when your mouth is on his dick. Don't you feel better when he lubes you up or you're vagina is really wet when he thrusts inside you? That's exactly how it is for him. Everything slides and moves just right with an erotic sensation. The best way to understand is to try it out on him and watch how he reacts.

Here are several ways to make your head game extra wet.

Lube – Lubes are perfect for this and there's a lot of different ones to choose from. The key is to get one that's safe to be consumed (ie. edible and flavored). This way you both enjoy the blowjob. He enjoys the feeling while you enjoy the taste.

The Right Kind Of Condiment – If you really want to make it tastier then add condiments to the recipe. You can start basic with cream, honey, maple syrup and chocolate syrup. For those who take eating dick seriously this one's for you.

Chewing Gum – Gum naturally increases saliva production for better digestion, whether you digest all of him is up to you. Use this biological hack to your advantage and chew some a few minutes before you give him head.

Deep Throating – Deep-throating stimulates your gag reflex which quickly produces a lot of salivae. Even though it might not feel that great on your part it's a pretty neat shortcut you can use.

ENTHUSIASM

Enthusiasm, in all things, makes for a better journey and satisfied destination. You can use this effective technique to increase your man's pleasure. The best part is he can do the same for you.

I'm sure you know how hot it is when a guy you really like is eager to rip your clothes off and make you his. It's the same feeling when your man is driven to eat you out with nothing holding him back. You feel desired, appreciated and even worshipped. Your partner feels the same way every time you rip his belt off, pull down his pants and slide him into your mouth without warning. It gives him an unparalleled level of arousal.

This translates to every aspect of your romantic and sex life. Transform simple pecks on his cheeks into passionate kisses. A mere hug should be a warm embrace, even pinning him down snuggly when he tries to escape. Don't wait for him to change sex positions, grab him and toss him into the position you want. Instead of just moaning, whisper in his ear what you want him to do to you.

How to Become the Greatest at Oral Sex 2: The Practical Guide will give you hundreds of examples of what to say to your man!

This initiative and enthusiasm speaks volumes about how you feel about him not just sexually but romantically too. Attacking his penis like you're possessed with passion will make the entire experience a lot more intense for him. It will make you seem active and genuinely interested in his pleasure. This will not only make him feel wanted and satisfied, it will show that you see sex as an exciting activity versus a dull routine chore.

VARIATION IS YOUR FRIEND

It might seem obvious but shaking up how, when and where you perform oral sex will easily spice up your love life. Applying variation will have him eager for more, always wondering what crazy thing you'll do next.

Men LOVE variety. They like to be treated to completely new and interesting things. Have you ever noticed how they keep jumping from one hobby or project to the next? The same routine every single day bores them. So if you use the same techniques every time you give them head they'll get tired of it pretty fast. How to Become The Greatest at Oral Sex Series is all about making sure this never happens. The purpose of it is not just to keep things fresh from week to week but all year round.

MAKE IT A SPECIAL OCCASION

Any man would love to get a blowjob every morning and every night, even sometimes between energy draining activities. But this would only end badly. Good things are best served in small random doses.

Let me explain why.

If you got to eat your favorite food all day, every day you will love it at first. The first week will seem like heaven. The second will feel like Neverland. But on the third things start to get weird. The more weeks pass, the less interested you are in it. You'll want to taste something new and experience completely different flavors and aromas. In the end, your favorite food will no longer be your favorite.

Giving your man head is the same. He's going to love the thought of getting a blowjob twice day at first. He'll definitely enjoy the first week. But as more days pass it won't be special anymore. It won't feel like a treat to him.

You can ensure this doesn't happen by creating balance in frequency. Not too often, but not too seldom either.

Depending on your sex drive this may be tricky to work out. Stuff like this usually boils down to personal preferences and desire. It can mean doing it twice a week instead of five times or once a day instead of every time you guys are alone. Find the balance and it'll work wonders.

9 EATING FOOD OFF THE BODY

7 Tips For Using Food In The Bedroom

When it comes down to it, food and sex have similar qualities. They're nourishing, sensual and have wide varieties. Each is good on its own and when you combine them they become even better. Foodplay is an interesting way to reinvent your sex life and ideal for long-term relationships.

"There are many benefits of monogamous relationships that couples enjoy with the primary being, sex-wise, they have the option to really explore each other's sexual nature," says Garrick Ruben, a matchmaker, and life coach. Since you've been together for a long time, both you and your partner know each other's tastes. It's very easy for you to express what you do and don't like individually. New experiences like this which involves incorporating new elements in a familiar act will strengthen the bonds between you.

Food and sex are both associated with biological needs as well as mental and emotional urges. We don't only do them because we're driven to but they also feel good.

"There's a primal, animalistic feel when eating and an unexplained hotness when licking our fingers," says Katie Waite, a sex and intimacy coach. "Our daily lives have strayed from the once welcome delectable nature of sex and food that enhanced now dull experiences. Food is a powerful medium for sexual metaphors that makes sex more seductive."

To get started using food in sex and foreplay make sure to properly divulge your medical backgrounds. This is to ensure that you get foods that you or your partner isn't allergic to. In addition to this, we have more tips below.

1. Keep it sweet and light.

If you're going to use food in sex you have to view it as an appetizer to the main course (sex). This means staying away from the savory or spicy type of foods. The sweeter the better.

Explore really sweet stuff like ice cream toppings. Health nuts can substitute artificial sweets with more natural ones like cherries and strawberries. If you want to have the best of both worlds, then use both in the bedroom.

The only warning we'll give you is not to eat too much. Though sugars provide us with energy, being overfull will slow you down and someone will fall asleep. If someone ends up asking for seconds, then it may mean it's actually lunch time.

2. Keep food away from your private parts.

Mixing food and private parts is a major No-no for a number of reasons. Firstly, there's a chance of infection or skin irritation in the area. Besides using plain ice with no extravagant additives, keep all food fun above the waist. There are a lot of erotic places up there too.

3. Engage all your senses.

Food is mainly for taste but we're going to go beyond that when we're using it in the bedroom. Explore other sense such as smell and touch. Experimenting with melting chocolate or take the temperature all the way down with flavored popsicles.

Gently run them over sensitive body parts like the neck, earlobes, nipples and lips. While you're doing this maintain action below the waist by stroking the parts where food is prohibited.

4. Get creative with your mouth.

Varying the amount of pressure and speed with your mouth is what will separate a good experience from a memorable one. It's good to lick food off his body but you can make it better by sucking it off his finger or nibbling it off his body (especially around the nipples). A little bit of teeth is fine once they're comfortable with it. You can also start with light gentle lip rubbing and then move on to swallow portions of his skin in your mouth – not like a cannibal of course.

5. Come prepared.

There's no way you'd go hiking without some food, a compass and a bottle of water, right? You should be equally prepared when you're going to start playing with food. Lay down some sheets or blankets you won't mind soiling. For clean-up, bring quick utensils such as napkins or baby wipes. Earlier we mentioned using chocolate, you can make distributing it easier and neater by using a drizzle bottle. In addition to all that keep the usual stuff nearby (condoms, lube, toys)

6. Have fun.

There's a reason most sexual stuff have the word 'play' in it, sex is all about having fun. Capitalize on your imagination when using food during sex with your partner. Make whipped cream crowns on his dick and then treat him like a king. He'll be baffled by your creativity and skills.

7. Clean each other off afterward.

Okay, so you've had a well-balanced meal of your partner and now it's time to wash up. Group together everything you've used during your dining experience so it's easy to deal with them later. Now it's time to jump into the shower and wash away all traces of your meal. The best thing about this part is that it might even lead to Dessert.

10 GOLDEN SHOWERS

Golden showers, commonly referred to as 'watersports', are sexual acts that incorporate urine. The lamer and more hard to remember medical term for urine fetish is urolagnia but you don't have to really use it even if it applies to you. "Golden showers" has a better ring to it.

Even though you might think this is pretty uncommon, PornHub reported a 287% increase in golden showers search related terms on January the 11th after Donald Trump was accused of experimenting with this kink himself.

We won't get too much into that but discovering someone else has an interest in such things means people are more open-minded than we initially thought. Realizing that the world is becoming more experimental in various ways is a welcomed phenomenon. Though the accusations mentioned he was using watersports to deface popular figures you can use golden showers for sexual satisfaction. If you've been interested in giving or receiving a golden shower, here's a simple guide on how to best get it done.

Golden showers: why are they a turn-on?

Golden showers are sexy to people for several reasons. Those who are into it usually associate the action with humiliation and so use it a lot in BDSM. Others typically just like watching their partner pee.

Besides peeing on each other, golden shower lovers engage in other activities like drinking each other's urine or playing tease and denial games. This could be things like allowing a partner to drink tons of water and dare them to hold their pee for as long as possible while the other partner performs sexual acts on them.

Golden showers: are they safe?

The mere fact that we've been flushing urine for a great portion of modern times will instinctively make us believe it's unhygienic to play with it. Urine, by itself, is very safe since it's sterile. The only way it can really do much harm is if someone ingests tons of chemical pollutants. Once they get past the thought of dying from touching or drinking urine, the next thing most people worry about is the smell. Urine can sometimes have a very strong smell if the person is dehydrated or drunk. You can easily avoid strong scents by drinking some water before you start.

The main things you would have to be mindful in terms of safety are:

1. Drinking. Drinking urine, whether yours or others, is generally safe. The only thing you should be cautious about is what part of the urine flow you should actually drink. The initial part of the urine, once it exits urethra, may contain bacteria from the surrounding area. To avoid this, simply allow the head of the flow to run off and catch the urine midstream.

2. Over-hydration. This usually isn't a problem for newbies but you can still take it into consideration. The danger comes from mixing power-play and piss-play since you can suffer from water intoxication. Yeah, that's a thing. You definitely need to be hydrated if you're going to mess around with golden showers but don't go too far.

Golden showers: location, location, location

Bathing in a golden shower on the porch would be hot but not a good idea. The most natural place to take your fetish is in the bathroom. Similar wet rooms like this are ideal since it makes the clean-up pretty easy. Besides, you probably pee in the shower already anyway. It's just going to be more fun this time.

Using wet rooms are encouraged but bedrooms are still a great playground. With just a few adjustments and extra materials, you can quickly transport your bedroom into a Golden Shower kingdom. To make sure that none of your furniture gets damaged or stained you can use special rubber or PVC sheets at an affordable cost. In the event you find these materials uncomfortable, the higher end alternatives like those made by Sheets of San Fransisco are fluid-proof while feeling like normal sheets. If you're planning to indulge in this fetish on a regular basis, then we recommend investing in these.

How do I tell my partner I'm into golden showers?

This is a tough one. Finding a way to somehow smoothly slip this topic into everyday conversation is not as easy as talking about what you want to have for dinner – unless you're discussing what to drink with it then you can insert it as a joke. But that's if you're really slick.

The easiest way to test the waters of this subject is to have them read a little bit of this book so that they understand it's not so unusual after all. A Channel 4 Great British Sex Survey that explored various sexual quirks and fetishes of thousands of people across the UK resulted in watersports making it into the top 10. That should be enough proof. Even if you're partner is still not interested at least you know you're not the only one who likes this stuff.

11 SHOWER SEX

More often than not sex is likely to happen in the shower even though there was no intention before you both got in there. Being wet makes everything ten times as sexy even though slippery showers can lead to fumbling and accidents. You know what kills the mood more than a surprise visit from your mom, ambulances and their annoying sirens. Other stuff, like your kid's toys, hurt more than help since they aren't the toys for such a situation.

Despite all the possible mishaps, showers are one of the best places to have sex and you should do it more. It's great for a quickie before work in the morning. If you haven't had much luck with shower sex then we'll help you master it. We've compiled a list of sexy oral, vaginal and anal positions you will enjoy in the shower.

Just in case you have second thoughts about kneeling in the hard shower you can place a towel under your knees so it's more comfortable. Additionally, if you're worried about being unable to bring your toys into the shower there are tons of waterproof versions you can use.

Wet Cowgirl/Cowboy

If your shower comes with a fairly big bathtub then this one will be easy for you. Have your partner sit in the bathtub with their legs stretched out. Now you can lower yourself on his hard shaft.

Soaked Standing Oral

While he's splashing water on his face why not give him a quick blowjob. Simply get on your knees and help him clean what's valuable to the both of you.

Standing Wet Doggy

Now switch it up and bend over under the shower head. From here he can thrust into from behind. If you need support use the walls or anything else that's stable enough.

The Shower Rim

If you've avoided rimming simply because down there may be a bit dirty, doing it in the shower solves that. Once you cleaned your ass crack, have your man sit on the edge of the bathtub and lick away.

Steamy Seated Peasant

Peasant is taken from Kama Sutra and it describes when a woman leans back into her partner's lap and opens her legs. From here it's easy to penetrate her vagina and play with her clit.

Since your shower's bathtub is a bit enclosed this position will be a bit snug. Even so, it makes for a very intimate experience that you can highlight with candle lights.

Hot Confessional

If you have a bench in your shower this one will be easy for you. If not, it means more towels might get wet since you'd have to stack them to get the same effect. Another alternative is sitting on the edge of the bathtub but that may still need a towel so your partner doesn't keel over.

Once you've got everything set up then the recipient of this blowjob would be sitting while the other is kneeling between their thighs. Now you can enjoy a wet steamy head.

12 FREAKY CAR SEX

1. Don't want to waste time getting undressed? Wear a short dress or skirt and crotchless panties under it so he has easy access.

2. Get your man ready for what's coming by stroking his dick through his pants. At the same time, go ahead and play with your clit too. You'll be wet and he'll be hard, so all you need to do is make him pull over and pull out.

3. Mirrors make sex even sexier and cars tend to have a lot. Utilize each one by positioning them perfectly to capture your bodies in motion.

4. We recommend keeping the windows up if you're in a public place like a fast food restaurant. But if you're far at the edge of the woods on a lonely road, roll down the windows and let your moans join the sounds of nature.

5. The easiest way to get business done is with you on top. Just avoid the driver's seat or the horn will give you a heart attack.

6. You might be far from the bedroom but that doesn't mean you can't use toys. Find what you can to make things more interesting.

7. Take your BDSM skills mobile by using the seatbelts as bondage. Keep him strapped in as you ride him like a mad horse.

8. After a while, you're gonna need to rest so lay on the back seat and let your man jump on top of you.

9. With your legs spread wide, it's pretty easy for him to go down on you. Don't pass up the opportunity.

10. If you want to get more creative, open the sunroof and stick your head out. While you're tanning in the sun you can sit on his face.

11. You know what's hot? Sucking his dick while he's cruising down a highway. Try not to distract him too much unless you wanna die with a dick in your mouth.

12. Step it up a notch and take things outside. Get on the hood of the car and let him have his way with you. Just make sure to visit a car wash to remove all the stains.

13. If you don't want to risk denting the car then use the hood as support as your man slams you from behind.

14. Having sex with ridiculous music blaring in the background will quickly ruin the mood. Make things even hotter by connecting your phone to the radio and playing all your sexy songs.

15. There's nothing wilder than doing it in the truck bed. Don't be afraid to join his other tools that are back there.

16. The closer it is to sunset the more intense the sex will be. You won't be preoccupied with looking out for strangers and when the stars pop out it'll be a romantic setting.

17. As your tongue massages his ear, whisper naughty lines to him so he has an even bigger erection. Just make sure it's not loud enough for pedestrians to join in on the fun.

18. Sexiness without practicality would lead to some awkward stuff. Make sure the A/C is on so your ass sweat doesn't get into his mouth when you're sitting on his face.

19. No matter where you do it, there's a guarantee that there are going to be more stains inside than out. Make sure you have a clean-up plan for when everything is done.

13 BDSM TIPS AND TRICKS

BDSM is the thing many people shy away from but are secretly into. It's a great way to spice up your love life and keep things interesting.

Sometimes we need to revisit how we operate in our intimate relationships. This is especially crucial for long-term relationships that have the potential of extending even longer. The virus of such relationships is complacency. Once it infects your beautiful romance, your love life will sour as affection quickly transforms into resentment. Many people think it is difficult or impossible but the reality of it will shock you.

Fortunately, humans being as inventive as they are, there are numerous ways to prevent such a calamity from happening at all. It is encouraged to keep the romance going by any means necessary but the physical aspect of things will need attention too. Nurturing both will lead to a relationship that satisfies "till death do us part".

Getting physical to keep the romance alive

No matter what people may say sex is vital in any loving and potentially long-lasting relationship. Of course, there will be those who believe differently and even claim that true love transcends sex but they will succumb to their urges soon enough. Especially in ways they don't expect. The truth is sex plays a crucial role in solidifying relationships, dissolving stress and tensions and also bringing a couple closer.

Even so, no matter how great the sex is, it can become dispassionate if you don't actively attempt to make it more interesting. This will echo through your entire relationship and cause it to deteriorate from all angles.

The 50 Shades of Play

To be honest, BDSM isn't for everyone. When it comes to sex most people stick to traditional routes. They tend to stay far away from anything that may seem unconventional. To really get into it and enjoy it, you must have a secret yearning for something unusual and experimental. You must be imaginative, open and trusting. If either one of you lacks these traits then that person will end up feeling awkward. Before you decide on what whips and ropes to buy you need to know what BDSM is first.

B stands for bondage. Bondage is basically applying restraints to your partner or to yourself. Some people get really aroused from not being able to resist someone forcing sex onto them. These people like the idea of being taken advantage of but safely with someone they know. How far you go with the restraints depends on personal preference and comfort level. How much control do they want to give up?

This can be anything in between being tied up with cloth and small ropes to extreme stuff like chains and handcuffs.

D represents domination. This is a specific type of role play where one partner is the dominator and the other is the dominated. The obvious distinction is that one gets to direct the sex scenes while the other submits to whatever is planned. The dominator usually has games prepared and dictates exactly what the other partner can and cannot do. They basically control the dominated.

SM is for sado-masochism. Put simply, SM utilizes pain in sexual activities. The sado half of the word refers to feeling pleasure from causing pain while masochism means getting pleasure from receiving pain. Much akin to bondage, SM has a wide spectrum of applications and can be very diverse in how extreme things are executed.

Biting, for example, is on the very tame side of the spectrum. This is where people usually start out along with gentle spanking and twisting nipples. In the middle, we have things like slapping, spanking, and whipping. As you get closer to the more extreme end you'll come across people incorporating painful contraptions from medieval times. It gets crazy real fast and if you aren't careful someone can get seriously hurt without the pleasure.

The next steps for trying out BDSM

We've already cautioned that BDSM isn't for everyone. Only a few people will be into the extreme nature of sex that BDSM explores. Though how deep you actually burrow into this form of sex is highly dependent on your personality. BDSM requires not only an open mind but also clear communication between the parties involved.

Next, you'll find some pointers that will guide you to have the right discussion with your partner before you dive into BDSM,

#1. Mutual interests- This is the first topic that would need to be covered when deliberating to incorporate BDSM into your lives. Do you both want this? Pitch the idea to your partner and pay keen attention to what they say and how they react. If they completely disagree then it's recommended that you accept and never revisit the topic again lest they feel bullied.

If you somehow manage to persuade them or if their mouth says yes and their body is giving a different signal, then this could lead to problems down the road. Your partner may only agree or get involved to make you satisfied. If you ever suspect this is happening, be sure to identify the signs and then discontinue the related activities immediately.

You would end up doing this to ensure that your relationship doesn't suffer from the other partner's discontent. The original aim of getting into this was to keep them enthusiastic, not chase them away. Preserve your relationship by knowing when to stop.

#2. Degrees of interest- Okay, so now you've gotten past the hardest part and your partner is interested. At this point, you need to examine that degree of interest and see how deep you both are willing to go. Do you want it to be done on special occasions, maybe once a month or do you want it to be a big part of your sex life?

The next thing is identifying the roles you'll both play especially when it comes to which aspect of BDSM you'll take part in. The last thing you want is your partner expecting a little spanking and he ends up blindfold in a makeshift dungeon with weapons that'll scar for life.

#3. Tools of the trade- Picking up from that you will need to discuss what kind of toys and tools you'll be using. Most BDSM toys are pretty gruesome and definitely not recommended for lightweights. It's all about starting simple and working your way up as you get comfortable. You guys can prepare beforehand on which toys you will buy for use so no-one gets a heart attack.

#4. Play it safe- Indulging in BDSM without a safe word is like begging for a trip to the emergency room followed by a psychiatrist. This word is usually used by the dominated or object of the sexual acts. When this word is uttered the fun should immediately stop without questions.

Since BDSM is all about enjoying a kind of forced sex it would be typical for a partner to yell "No!" or "Stop!" so these words shouldn't be used. Try words that are completely off topic and unusual. You can even make up your own words to keep it unique. Whatever it is, just don't forget it!

#5. The community- The BDSM community is insanely active and loves entertaining newcomers. It's a great place for tips and advice since most people are pretty experienced in what they're doing. You can use the chats and forums to discuss interests or plan meet-ups. It's good to be a part of a community that supports what you find to be exciting. Don't be afraid to reach out and connect with others.

ABOUT THE AUTHOR

Amazon's International Bestselling Author Jessica King is the Author of the International #1 Bestseller "How to Become the Greatest at Oral Sex: Sex Secrets that puts a Spell on Him." She was once your typical clumsy, awkward chick, always falling for the wrong guys. Being used, abused and taken for a complete idiot in the past, until she stumbled upon a "great secret" that dramatically changed her life.

She has been sharpening her craft for years and after a decade she has decided to share this secret in a simple "easy to read" manual—intended to help women and even men around the world—that has sold thousands of copies in the United States, United Kingdom, Europe and Canada with copies sold in Australia, India, Mexico, and the Caribbean.

Jessica has learned that different cults, religions, sects, groups, secret societies and fraternal orders all have one thing in common: The Mind & the Power of Belief. The simple secrets and techniques her book contain has expanded readers consciousness and resonated with their souls, making it an Amazon Favorite.

36073418R00042

Made in the USA
Lexington, KY
11 April 2019